FAST FACTS

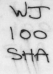

Urinary Continence

Second edition

Indispens
Guides to
Clinical
Practice

Julian Shah

Senior Lecturer, Institute of Urology and
Nephrology, University College, London;
Consultant Urologist at St Peter's Hospital
and the Middlesex Hospital, London, and
the Spinal Injuries Unit, Royal National
Orthopaedic Hospital Trust, Stanmore, UK

Gary Leach

Director, Tower Urology Institute for
Continence, Cedars-Sinai Medical Center,
and Clinical Professor of Urology,
University of Southern California,
Los Angeles, California, USA

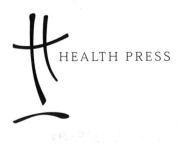

HEALTH PRESS

Oxford

Fast Facts – Urinary Continence
First published 1998
Second edition 2001

The publisher and the authors have made every effort to ensure the
accuracy of this book, but cannot accept responsibility for any errors or
omissions.

The publication of this book has been supported through an unrestricted
educational grant from Pharmacia & Upjohn.

The views expressed in this publication are those of the authors and not
necessarily those of Pharmacia & Upjohn.

A CIP catalogue record for this title is available from the British Library.

ISBN 1-899541-64-0

Shah, J (Julian)
Fast Facts – Urinary Continence/
Julian Shah, Gary Leach

Printed by Fine Print (Services) Ltd, Oxford, UK.

Glossary

CISC: clean intermittent self-catheterization involves passing a catheter into the bladder to remove urine when the patient cannot pass urine normally. The procedure, which is not usually carried out under sterile conditions, is performed by the patient or a carer every few hours during the day and sometimes at night

CLAM: augmentation ileocystoplasty increases the size of the abnormal bladder by attaching an opened segment of ileum or colon

CMG: a cystometrogram measures the pressure in the bladder during filling and emptying

DI: detrusor instability is uninitiated detrusor contractions during bladder filling giving rise to the sensation of frequency of micturition and urgency

DSD: detrusor sphincter dyssynergia is uncoordinated external sphincter contractions during bladder contraction giving rise to obstructed voiding seen in neurological bladder dysfunction

EBNS: endoscopic bladder neck suspension is an operation in which the bladder neck and urethra are supported by sutures placed on either side of the bladder neck and suspended from the rectus sheath or by bone fixation

ES: the external striated sphincter is the voluntarily controlled external sphincter mechanism, which is partly responsible for urinary continence

DH: detrusor hyperreflexia is abnormal detrusor contractions seen during bladder filling in association with neuropathy

GSI: genuine stress incontinence is the involuntary leakage of urine associated with a rise in intra-abdominal pressure due to weakness of the external striated sphincter mechanism

IDSO: isolated distal sphincter obstruction is the failure of the external sphincter to relax, giving rise to the outflow obstruction seen in certain forms of neuropathy

PMD: post-micturition dribbling is the leakage of urine after micturition has been completed and is most commonly seen in men

RU: the residual urine is the urine left behind in the bladder after the completion of micturition

Strangury: severe pain in the urethra associated with an intense desire to pass urine

SWI: sphincter weakness incontinence is incontinence due to weakness of the external striated sphincter – see GSI

TD: terminal dribbling is dribbling towards the end of micturition seen in association with decompensation of the detrusor in outflow obstruction

VCUG: a videocystourogram consists of cystometry in conjunction with radiological screening of the bladder

smoothly and rapidly leaving no urine behind in the bladder. Investigation of the process of micturition is known as urodynamics.

Although babies and infants have 'urinary incontinence' for which they wear nappies/diapers, this is not abnormal voiding. The bladder emptying that takes place at an early age is the result of cortically evoked coordinated detrusor function with appropriate external sphincter relaxation leading to rapid bladder emptying though residual urine may be left. It is the development of social awareness that makes small children subsequently able to void in suitable places.

Urinary incontinence may be defined as the involuntary loss of urine. A number of different clinical problems that affect the ability of the bladder to store urine can lead to urinary incontinence. Any dysfunction of the neurology, anatomy or physiology of the bladder may give rise to a disorder in urine storage and/or to abnormal voiding with or without urinary incontinence. Abnormal voiding may present as high-pressure obstruction, low-pressure/slow flow or urinary retention. Urinary incontinence may occur as a result of obstructed voiding either because of the associated detrusor instability (DI) that may develop or chronic retention with overflow. Thus incontinence can occur in association with a variety of conditions that affect bladder function, which will require correction without the need for enhancing the bladder outflow. Urinary incontinence is associated with:

- weakness of the urinary outlet – genuine stress incontinence (GSI)
- failure of the bladder to store urine due to high bladder pressure – urge incontinence
- a combination of weakness of the urinary outlet and failure of the bladder to store urine – mixed incontinence (urge and stress incontinence)
- a bladder that is overfull and overflows (chronic retention) – overflow incontinence
- abnormal communications of the urinary tract (e.g. a fistula).

Risk factors for urinary incontinence

Age. Urinary incontinence occurs in infancy and childhood due to immaturity of the nervous system. By the age of 2–3 years, most children are able to appreciate the need to void and learn to do so in the appropriate setting. However, bed-wetting may persist until the age of 6 years before it

TABLE 1.1

Prevalence of urinary incontinence in the UK

Age (years)	Women (%)	Men (%)
5–14	5.1	6.9
15–24	4.0	1.4
25–34	5.5	0.8
35–44	16.1	2.4
45–54	16.6	5.5
55–64	16.7	5.7
65–74	14.1	12.1
> 75	18.0	15.4

becomes clinically significant (see page 38). In the elderly, urinary incontinence is most often due to abnormalities of detrusor function, with DI being the most common cause.

Gender. Urinary incontinence is more common in women than in men (Table 1.1). Women are more likely to develop stress incontinence due to weakening of the pelvic floor and ES as a consequence of childbirth and ageing. In men, the development of stress incontinence tends to relate to prostatectomy and neurological dysfunction. The incidence of urinary incontinence among elderly men receiving diuretic therapy is said to be the same as that among elderly women.

Obesity itself is not thought to cause urinary incontinence and does not appear to influence the outcome of surgery.

CHAPTER 2

Investigations and diagnosis

A detailed clinical history is essential in order to obtain an accurate diagnosis in any patient with urinary incontinence. Using a proforma (Figure 2.1) to record the clinical symptoms and the results of the examination will assist the diagnosis, and indicate the investigations needed.

Name: DOB: Age:

Address:

Tel - Home: Work: Occupation:

GP: Referred by:

                                               Date:

Frequency   Presenting Complaint

Nocturia

Urgency

Incontinence:

     Stress

     Urge

     Continuous/unconscious

     Pads – type and number

Hesitancy

Stream: normal/reduced/intermittent/variable

Terminal dribbling/post-micturition dribbling

Bladder emptying - complete/incomplete

Straining

Dysuria/infection/haematuria/strangury

Pain-renal/bladder/urethral/testicular/other

Sexual function

Past medical history

Family history

Drugs: Allergies

Examination: Diagnosis:

Rectal: prostate:normal/abnormal/size:

Vaginal: cystocele/rectocele/enterocele

   stress leak

   bimanual

   urethral position/mobility

Figure 2.1 Proforma for taking a detailed clinical history from patients with urinary incontinence and voiding dysfunction.

Lower urinary tract symptoms (LUTS) is the generic description for symptoms of bladder dysfunction. The symptoms of urinary incontinence may be divided into:

- irritative/urge syndrome
- obstructive/overflow
- post-micturition dribble (PMD)
- continuous incontinence
- GSI
- mixed incontinence
- nocturnal enuresis.

Irritative/urge syndrome

Irritative symptoms are the most common symptoms in patients with urinary incontinence.

Frequency of micturition may be defined as the passing of urine more than seven times during a 24-hour period. The number of times a person urinates during the day will of course be influenced by fluid intake, but assuming an average daily fluid intake of 1500–2000 ml/day, passing urine up to seven times can be considered normal. The average void is 200–300 ml, with the largest void usually being the first of the day after waking.

Nocturia is defined as being awoken by the desire to void. It is a common clinical complaint, especially in elderly patients. It has many causes, which are not necessarily due to bladder dysfunction (Table 2.1).

As a person ages, changes in the homeostatic mechanisms controlling urine production mean that more urine tends to be passed during the night than before, and this is probably the most common reason for nocturia. Physiological nocturia should not, however, be confused with other causes of nocturia. Peripheral oedema seen in the elderly or patients with immobility or cardiovascular disease is a common cause of nocturia.

Urgency is the urgent desire to void. A need to void immediately, or a feeling of impending incontinence, tends to signify detrusor overactivity. Urgency may, however, be associated with pain in the suprapubic region or urethra, and this is likely to signify hypersensitive bladder dysfunction.

TABLE 2.1
Causes of nocturia

Associated with ageing

- Loss of diurnal regulation of urine output (commonly seen in the elderly and in childhood enuresis)
- Peripheral oedema (due to inactivity, limb dependency and heart failure)

Specific causes

- Detrusor overactivity with or without obstruction
- Chronic retention of urine with overflow
- Excessive fluid intake
- Prostatic outflow obstruction due to benign prostatic hyperplasia or carcinoma
- Drugs (e.g. diuretics taken in the evening)
- Insomnia

Urge incontinence is leakage of urine that occurs inadvertently when a patient is trying not to void. The patient will feel an urgent desire to pass urine and may leak urine on the journey to the toilet. This usually takes the form of a few drops of urine leaking out before the patient arrives at the toilet, but some patients will void completely, especially those with detrusor hyperreflexia.

GSI is the involuntary loss of urine associated with a rise in intra-abdominal pressure without a significant change in bladder (detrusor) pressure (i.e. a stable bladder).

Mixed incontinence is the presence of both GSI and DI. These can combine to cause incontinence (combined incontinence) or each factor can cause incontinence at different times, for example, with urgency, change in posture, and leakage with coughing and sneezing.

Nocturnal enuresis is incontinence during sleep and generally occurs in children. It may occur alone (DI < 25%) or in association with daytime symptoms of urinary frequency and urgency when bladder instability is often present (75% of cases).

Obstructive symptoms

The cardinal symptoms of obstruction are:

- hesitancy
- poor stream
- stop-start micturition
- terminal dribbling
- feeling of incomplete emptying/retention of urine.

Straining to pass urine is unusual with prostatic outflow obstruction, but is associated with urethral strictures or stenosis, and detrusor hypocontractility or acontractility. Women strain to pass urine more commonly than men as a result of poor detrusor contractility. In men, straining is usually associated with urethral strictures or a 'decompensated' bladder.

Post-micturition dribble

PMD can present in males of any age and consists of leakage of urine after micturition when the penis has been placed back into the underclothes. Approximately 80% of the male population suffer with this symptom. PMD, which causes soiling of the underclothes and sometimes even the outer clothing, is due to the leakage of a few drops of urine that pool in the bulbar urethra after micturition has been completed and drain due to gravity some moments later. PMD is seldom associated with clinical abnormalities and may be avoided either by waiting until the remaining urethral urine has been passed, or by compression of the bulbar urethra in the perineum and milking of the penile urethra at the end of micturition. Urethral stricture or diverticulum may be rare causes of PMD. If voiding dysfunction is present, flowmetry should be the first investigation.

Continuous incontinence

The continuous loss of urine tends to be associated with urinary tract fistulae or with chronic retention with overflow, which occurs most commonly in men with obstruction caused by an enlarged prostate.

Unconscious incontinence

Some patients are unaware of urinary loss. The loss is noticed only when the patient discovers wet underclothes or pads, or when the patient finds urine running down the thigh. In general, patients with neurological dysfunction may experience this type of incontinence because of loss of awareness of bladder fullness and the need to void, loss of sensation in the perineum or severe sphincter weakness incontinence (intrinsic sphincter deficiency, or ISD).

Other symptoms associated with incontinence

Inflammatory symptoms. Dysuria and strangury are both symptoms that may occur, along with urinary incontinence, as a result of inflammatory conditions (e.g. infection of the urinary tract, bladder calculi, bladder tumours or hypersensitivity of the urethra). These symptoms also occur in men with prostatitis, whether or not this is associated with abnormal bacteriological culture.

Haematuria may occur in an incontinent patient and should always be fully investigated. In these circumstances, although an associated underlying cause, such as infection, calculus or trauma from a catheter, is most likely, a bladder tumour or other urinary tract neoplasm may be present.

Physical examination

A physical and neurological examination should be carried out in all patients with urinary incontinence. Most neurological abnormalities that are associated with urinary incontinence will be obvious when the patient first presents. General neurological abnormalities, such as spinal cord injury (and the level of the injury), spina bifida, multiple sclerosis and parkinsonism, should also be recorded. Additional information that should be gained from the clinical examination includes:

- cerebral function
- sensory level
- muscular tone and power
- reflex activity
- spinal deformity
- skin dimple over lumbosacral area
- perianal sensation – reduced or absent
- anal tone and anal wink reflex
- bulbo-cavernosus reflex.

The suprapubic area should be palpated to see if the bladder is enlarged and percussed if the bladder is not easily palpated. Occasionally, the enlargement of the bladder is readily apparent (Figure 2.2).

Genital examination is essential. In women, the urethra should be examined and the patient asked to cough repeatedly (at least six coughs) to demonstrate the presence or absence of stress incontinence. The appearance of the vagina, the presence or absence of atrophic vaginitis, urethral hypermobility, cystocele, rectocele, vault prolapse, enterocele and uterine prolapse should all be noted; it may be necessary to examine the patient in the standing position to detect incontinence and vaginal prolapse. In the male patient, the appearance of the prepuce and external meatus may be a guide to distal urethral causes of voiding difficulties or PMD, which appear to the patient as urinary incontinence, yet may be due to phimosis, meatal stenosis or distal urethral stenosis. Digital rectal examination should also be performed in all men to assess the size and consistency of the prostate, and to detect any abnormality suggestive of carcinoma.

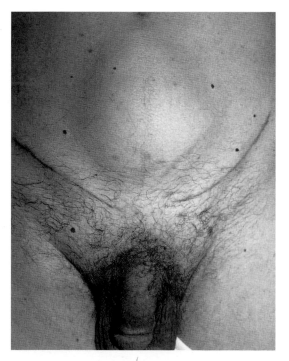

Figure 2.2
In patients with chronic retention of urine, the bladder is often grossly enlarged.

Investigations

Further investigation (Figure 2.3) is usually necessary to confirm a diagnosis of urinary incontinence, but the tests undertaken will depend, to some extent, on the facilities available. Nevertheless, the general principle for investigating incontinence must be to gain as much information as possible so that an accurate diagnosis can be made.

Frequency/volume voided chart. This will provide useful information about bladder function and the degree of incontinence (Figure 2.4). Factors that may be identified from a frequency/volume voided chart include:
- 'over-drinking' by patients who drink large volumes of fluid during the day either from habit or following medical advice
- variations in fluid intake that produce troublesome urinary symptoms at particular times in the day
- regular voiding of small volumes of urine, which is characteristic of patients who suffer from frequency of micturition; volumes of 25–150 ml indicate an abnormality of bladder function due to either reduced bladder capacity or DI
- the frequency of nocturnal enuresis.

A frequency/volume voided chart is also useful to assess and monitor treatment, and to demonstrate the benefits of treatment to the patient.

Urine culture. The urine should be examined for blood and reducing substances by dipstick testing, and a midstream specimen of urine (MSU) should be obtained from all patients with urinary incontinence to exclude the possibility of infection or inflammation. In addition, microscopic examination of the urine should be performed to determine whether any red or white blood cells are present.

Urine cytology should be performed in the presence of incontinence and haematuria or when red cells are seen on urine microscopy to exclude urothelial neoplasia, and particularly in patients over 50 years of age with irritative symptoms.

Imaging investigations may be necessary in certain specific situations.

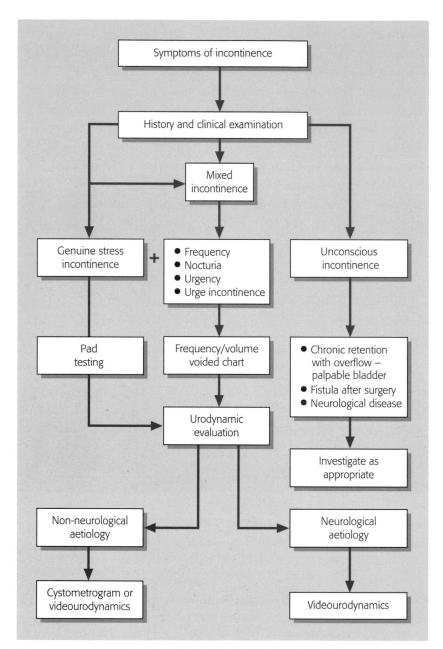

Figure 2.3 Recommendations for the investigation of a patient with incontinence; if particular investigations are not readily available, advice from a urologist should be sought.

FREQUENCY / VOLUME CHART

Name.................................   Record Number.............................

Date of Start................

	Sunday		Monday		Tuesday		Wednesday		Thursday		Friday		Saturday	
Day in Cycle														
	IN	OUT	IN	OUT	IN	OUT	IN	OUT	IN	OUT	IN	OUT	IN	OUT
09.00 - 10.00														
10.00 - 11.00														
11.00 - 12.00														
12.00 - 13.00														
13.00 - 14.00														
14.00 - 15.00														
15.00 - 16.00														
16.00 - 17.00														
17.00 - 18.00														
18.00 - 19.00														
19.00 - 20.00														
20.00 - 21.00														
21.00 - 22.00														
22.00 - 23.00														
23.00 - 24.00														
24.00 - 01.00														
01.00 - 02.00														
02.00 - 03.00														
03.00 - 04.00														
04.00 - 05.00														
05.00 - 06.00														
06.00 - 07.00														
07.00 - 08.00														
08.00 - 09.00														
WAKING														
RETIRING														

Enter amount drank in the "in" column.
Enter volumes of urine passed in the "out" column.
Please return this completed chart at your next visit.

Figure 2.4 The frequency/volume voided chart is a simple method of highlighting abnormal fluid intake and increased frequency of micturition.

Plain radiography. A preliminary plain abdominal radiograph may be performed to look for calculi and soft tissue masses in patients with a suspected urological abnormality. This is followed with urinary tract ultrasonography.

Ultrasonography is a sensitive method of detecting abnormalities of the kidneys. Renal scarring, calculi, dilatation and tumours may be sensitively picked up by this method. Scanning the bladder for residual urine, bladder wall thickness and calculi will aid both diagnosis and management.

Intravenous urography is used less commonly nowadays, having been replaced by ultrasonography for routine investigation. If, however, the ultrasound examination suggests renal obstruction or there is leakage from a fistula, intravenous urography may be appropriate.

Urodynamic investigations. Incontinence usually results from a change in the dynamics of the bladder and urinary sphincters, which will be identified by urodynamic investigations.

Uroflowmetry. Measurement of the urine flow rate (Figure 2.5) is a simple test, which should be performed in all patients with voiding dysfunction and incontinence. The patient should be asked to void with a comfortably full bladder in relaxed surroundings. A voided volume of at least 150–200 ml is necessary for the flow rate to be interpreted properly; many elderly patients do not void more than 150 ml at each void and this may influence the results of the test. It must be remembered, however, that variations in flow rates do occur and a single test should not be used as the basis of a firm clinical diagnosis. The flow-rate clinic in which three flow rates are obtained produces the most useful information.

Subsequent measurement of the post-void residual urine by either ultrasonography or catheterization provides further information about the nature of bladder emptying.

Urodynamic testing takes 20–30 minutes. Patients, particularly men, will experience some discomfort during catheterization and a sympathetic approach by the clinician will make a significant difference to the success of the test. Vasovagal attacks, leading to fainting, can occur during the investigation, especially in younger men. Patients may suffer some burning urethral discomfort for up to 24 hours after the test, but this can be minimized by increasing the fluid intake during this period. The incidence of culture-proven urinary tract infection after urodynamics is only 1%, but patients at higher risk of infection (i.e. with indwelling catheters, chronic residual urine, prostatitis or neurological dysfunction) should be given antibiotic prophylaxis.

Normal voiding

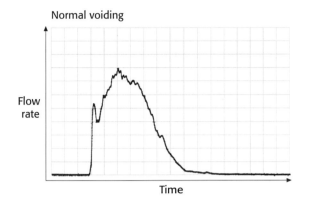

Reduced flow rate in prostatic outflow obstruction

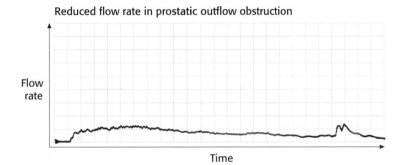

Intermittent flow rate in a patient straining to void

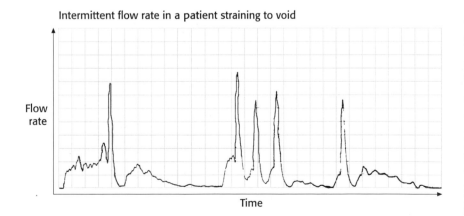

Figure 2.5 The urine flow rate can indicate a number of abnormalities and should be performed in all patients with voiding dysfunction and incontinence.

Cystometry assesses the normal bladder cycle of filling and pressure/flow analysis evaluates bladder emptying. It involves the measurement of bladder pressures during both filling and emptying, the urine flow rate and the presence or absence of residual urine. The bladder is filled with saline at room temperature via a small bore (10 Ch or smaller) urethral catheter and bladder pressure measured via a 4 Ch catheter passed alongside the filling catheter. The pressure in the rectum is recorded simultaneously to identify artefactual pressure rises resulting from coughing, talking, straining and

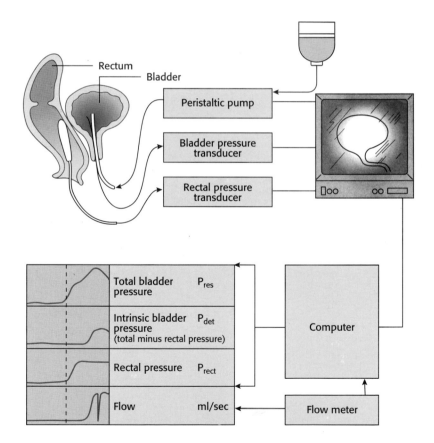

Figure 2.6 Cystometry measures bladder pressures during both filling and emptying. Measurement of the rectal pressure enables artefactual pressure rises to be identified.

changing position, which would adversely affect the interpretation of the intravesical pressure changes (Figure 2.6).

Although filling cystometry is of course unphysiological, the normal bladder may be filled at a rapid rate without any change in pressure. By filling the bladder at different rates according to the nature of the suspected bladder dysfunction, cystometry can be used to elicit any underlying abnormality.

- Fast-fill cystometry, at a rate of 100 ml/minute, is intended to provoke any underlying detrusor dysfunction, especially DI. Additional provocative tests such as coughing, changes in posture and bouncing up and down on the heels may uncover DI that was not apparent during rapid filling of the bladder.
- Medium-fill cystometry, at a rate of 30–60 ml/minute, may be used as an alternative to fast filling, particularly in patients known to have hypersensitive bladders, which are associated with urinary frequency, nocturia and pain.
- Slow-fill cystometry, at a rate of 10–20 ml/minute, is recommended in patients known to suffer from DI or detrusor hyperreflexia, or when the bladder is suspected to be poorly compliant (Figure 2.7). Slow-fill cystometry is intended to mimic natural slow filling. It reduces the likelihood of bladder contractions developing too early in the filling part of the test, which could give rise to incontinence before useful information is obtained about the ability of the bladder to store urine. If a bladder contracts too early during the filling phase because bladder filling was too rapid, much of the benefit of the test may be lost.

Videourodynamics, which combines cystometry using a contrast medium with simultaneous radiological screening of the bladder and urethra, is currently the gold standard of urodynamic investigation (Figure 2.8). It provides information about the appearance of the bladder, urethra, sphincters and reflux into the ureters, and is more helpful in the diagnosis of complex cases of incontinence than cystometry alone. Simultaneous video recording of the screening process is also useful for data interpretation, as well as for teaching and research purposes.

Ambulatory urodynamics are helpful in the diagnosis of more complex cases, though it is not performed routinely in the USA. When the cause of

(a)

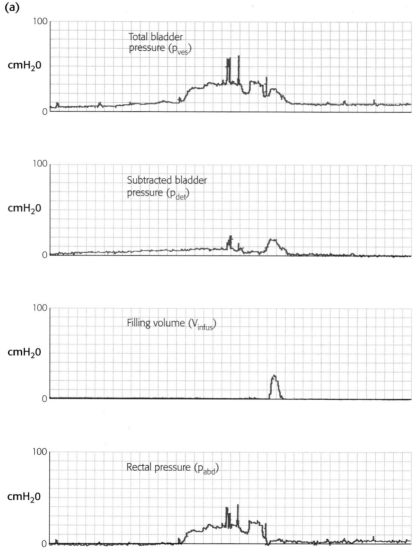

Figure 2.7 Cystometry demonstrating (a) a normal bladder and (b) (facing page) poor bladder compliance during filling in a patient with neuropathy. Bladder pressure rises steadily (*) to 40 cmH$_2$O, above the upper limit of normal of 15 cmH$_2$O. The wavy nature of the rectal pressure recording is due to rectal contractions.

(b)

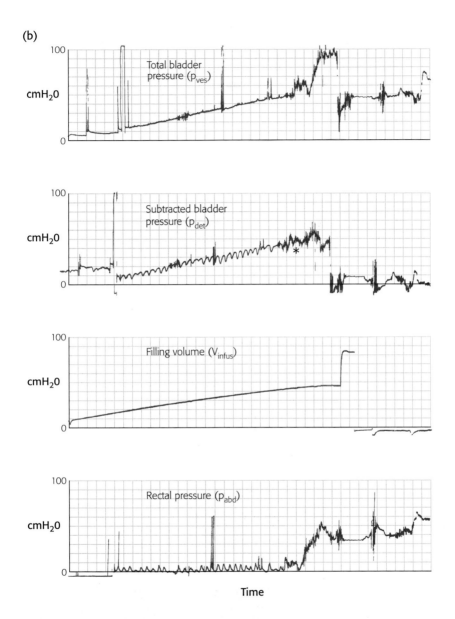

Time

incontinence is not determined by standard urodynamic techniques, ambulatory urodynamics may give a more sensitive assessment of urodynamic function, particularly when combined with a pad test for incontinence. However, problems with artefacts that occur during prolonged

25

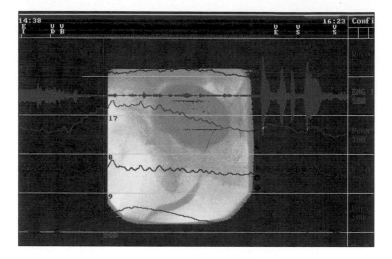

Figure 2.8 A videourodynamic study in a patient with prostatic outflow obstruction. The study shows the attenuated prostatic urethra (pink) with raised pressure (green) and low flow.

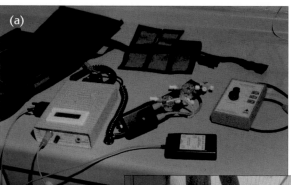

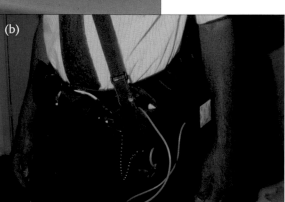

Figure 2.9
(a) Equipment needed for ambulatory urodynamics; (b) a patient undergoing ambulatory urodynamics testing.

recordings of this sort may make interpretation of the results more difficult. These studies should be available in specialized centres.

The patient is connected to an external computer box (Figure 2.9) via bladder and rectal catheters, as for standard urodynamics. The patient is able to indicate the normal sensation of bladder filling, urgency and incontinence via a patient control unit. Voiding may take place into a flow chamber in the urodynamic unit. The test is usually conducted over a duration of 4–6 hours or longer, or overnight for patients with nocturnal enuresis.

CHAPTER 3

Detrusor instability

Detrusor instability is defined by the International Continence Society as the occurrence of uninitiated detrusor contractions during bladder filling while the patient is attempting to inhibit the desire to void (Figure 3.1). Detrusor contractions below the norm of 15 cmH$_2$O are clinically significant if associated with the symptoms of frequency, nocturia and urgency, or micturition. It is thought that incidentally discovered DI may occur in up to 10% of normal individuals without giving rise to symptoms of incontinence.

DI gives rise to the frequency/urgency syndrome, which is associated with the symptoms of frequency, nocturia, urgency and urge incontinence (Table 3.1). The aetiology of DI may be:
- idiopathic, in which uninhibited detrusor contractions occur in a neurologically normal individual
- obstructive, which is seen most commonly in association with bladder outlet obstruction (i.e. prostatic obstruction and urethral strictures in men and urethral stenosis in women or after surgery for incontinence)

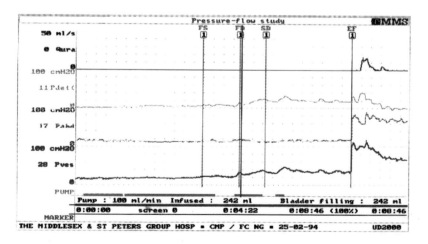

Figure 3.1 Cystometrogram from a patient with detrusor instability. The trace shows uninitiated detrusor contractions (∗) that exert a pressure greater than 15 cmH$_2$O during bladder filling while the patient is inhibiting the desire to void.

TABLE 3.1

Incidence of presenting symptoms in patients with detrusor instability

Symptom	Incidence (%)
Frequency	90
Nocturia	90
Urgency	78
Urge incontinence	86 in women
Stress incontinence	76 in women

- the result of detrusor hyperreflexia, in which uninitiated detrusor contractions occur in the presence of an underlying neuropathy (e.g. multiple sclerosis, spinal cord injury and spina bifida).

Some patients may present with symptoms suggestive of DI, but without any urodynamic abnormality. In such cases, a diagnosis of sensory urgency may be made and a cause sought.

Investigation of detrusor instability

Although the symptoms often point to detrusor dysfunction, sensory causes, such as infection, should be excluded by urine culture. A frequency/volume voided chart that shows irregular small-volume voids indicates bladder storage dysfunction.

Urodynamic investigation is the mainstay of diagnosis, but only approximately 50% of patients can be diagnosed using routine filling cystometry. Furthermore, additional provocative procedures during cystometry, such as coughing, changes in posture and heel jouncing (bouncing up and down on the heels), may help to reveal DI. A very fast flow rate may be seen in patients with enuresis due to a strong bladder, which can indicate pre-existing, but now resolved, bladder instability. Powerful after-contractions at the completion of voiding may be seen in patients with an underlying instability. If the symptoms indicate DI, but this is not demonstrated on routine filling cystometry, ambulatory urodynamic studies over a period of 4–6 hours will often reveal the detrusor dysfunction.

Management

Behavioural therapy involves demonstrating the presence of detrusor contractions to the patient, usually by visual means (e.g. a traffic light system or audible signal). The patient is connected to the urodynamic equipment as for cystometry (see page 22). When an abnormal contraction develops, a warning red light or sound is triggered. The patient is asked to inhibit the contraction thus changing the red light signal to green or stopping the sound output. This technique helps the patient not only to understand the abnormality causing the incontinence, but also provides effective treatment as long as the patient is prepared to maintain such a programme at home (without the equipment!).

Up to 60% of patients may show an improvement in symptoms, though urodynamic stability does not usually occur. However, follow up in an out-patient clinic is essential to help to motivate patients to learn to control their symptoms. Without reinforcement, the majority of patients will continue to suffer.

In a controlled trial, acupuncture cured symptoms over a relatively short period of follow up in 77% of patients with DI, though urodynamic parameters were unchanged.

Bladder training is an effective treatment for DI in many motivated patients. The patient is asked to delay micturition for increasing periods by inhibiting the desire to void. This technique, which was popularized by Frewen and is often known as the Frewen regimen, improves symptoms in many patients. Frewen reported that 75% of his patients were 'cured' of their symptoms after a 2-week period of in-patient bladder training. However, when these patients returned home, they tended to relapse as they were unable to maintain the regimen.

Changes in lifestyle that may lead to improvements in bladder dysfunction include:
- fluid restriction, after examination of the frequency/volume voided chart
- timed voiding
- eliminating stimulants, such as coffee, tea and alcohol, from the diet.

Pharmacological therapy. Anticholinergic drugs are the mainstay of treatment for detrusor instability.

- Oxybutynin, 2.5–5 mg three times daily, has a direct effect on the smooth muscle of the bladder as well as blocking the muscarinic effects of acetylcholine. Sustained-release oxybutynin is now available. It has a reduced side-effect profile, and doses can therefore be increased to 10–30 mg daily.

- Tolterodine is an effective anticholinergic agent and its selectivity for the bladder results in a low side-effect profile, particularly in terms of dry mouth. The recommended dose is 2 mg twice daily.

- Propiverine provides similar benefits to the other agents at a dose of 15 mg three times daily. It is not available in the USA.

- Imipramine, 10–25 mg three times daily, is an effective antidepressant and also has anticholinergic activity. It is particularly useful in children and the elderly.

- Propantheline bromide, 15 mg three times daily, has been available for many years and is a useful anticholinergic agent for the treatment of detrusor instability, though with the major anticholinergic side-effects.

Treatment should be given for at least 2 weeks in the first instance, but if the anticholinergic side-effects (e.g. dry mouth, blurred vision) are tolerable and symptoms have improved, the treatment may be continued indefinitely. If symptoms have not improved sufficiently, then the treatment dose may be increased. If symptoms still do not improve, then the medication should be changed to another drug or a combination of drugs, using any of the above. Most recently, long-acting oxybutynin has reduced the side-effect profile, making this effective medication more tolerable than immediate-release oxybutynin.

A number of new medications (e.g. darifenacin, trospium chloride) for the treatment of DI are currently undergoing clinical trials. These drugs may become available within the next 1–2 years and should reduce the incidence of side-effects that limit patient tolerance.

For patients using clean intermittent self-catheterization (CISC), intravesical oxybutynin has the benefit of improving bladder function with minimal anticholinergic side-effects. Oxybutynin, 5 mg in 30 ml saline, is instilled into the bladder at 8-hourly intervals after the bladder has been emptied; the saline should be as close to body temperature as possible and should be injected slowly, as some patients find that rapid injection of the fluid is associated with leakage. Oxybutynin instillation is not yet licensed.

In elderly women with atrophic vaginitis and urge or stress incontinence, oestrogen replacement therapy may be of benefit.

Intravesical agents. Oxbutynin is effective in reducing detrusor overactivity when instilled into the bladder three times a day in conjunction with intermittent catheterization. Capsaicin, an extract from chilli peppers, interferes with C fibres in the bladder wall and is used to reduce detrusor contractility in patients with multiple sclerosis. Resiniferotoxin is more effective than capsaicin but is still under investigation.

Neuromodulation is a new innovation in the treatment of incontinence. Sacral segmental (S_3) nerve stimulation with an electrode implanted via the S_3 foramen produces inhibition of detrusor instability. SANS™ (Stoller Afferent Nerve Stimulator; Urosurge, Inc., Coralville, IA, USA) is minimally

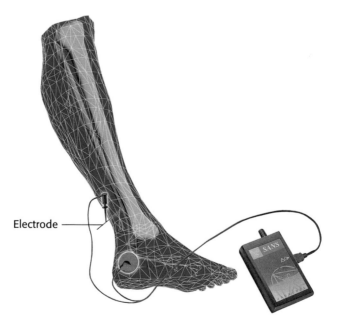

Electrode

Figure 3.2 In SANS™, an electrode is positioned near the ankle and treatment applied for 30 minutes each week. Reproduced with permission from UroSurge, Inc.

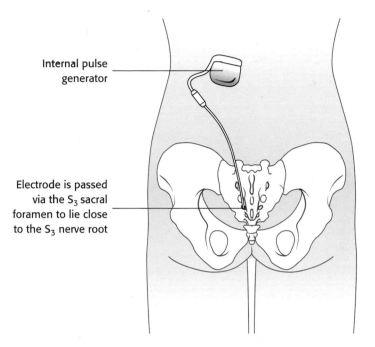

Internal pulse generator

Electrode is passed via the S_3 sacral foramen to lie close to the S_3 nerve root

Figure 3.3 In Interstim® therapy, a lead is placed near the left S_3 foramen and the internal pulse generator implanted to provide mild electrical stimulation to the sacral nerves that control the bladder, sphincter and pelvic floor muscles.

invasive, with the sacral nerve junction accessed via a nerve bundle near the ankle (Figure 3.2). It is still at an investigational stage and is not yet approved in the USA. An alternative system is Interstim® Therapy, Sacral Nerve Stimulation (Medtronic, Minneapolis, MN, USA) (Figure 3.3). Following an initial test in the patient, a lead, which is connected to an internal pulse generator, is placed near to S_3 sacral nerve under general anaesthetic. Side-effects appear to be minimal.

Surgery. Some patients find drug treatment intolerable because of the side-effects, or do not wish to take such treatment. Others would prefer a more permanent solution, such as that provided by surgery.

Cystodistension may temporarily help in minor degrees of bladder instability. However, most of the surgical procedures that have been used to

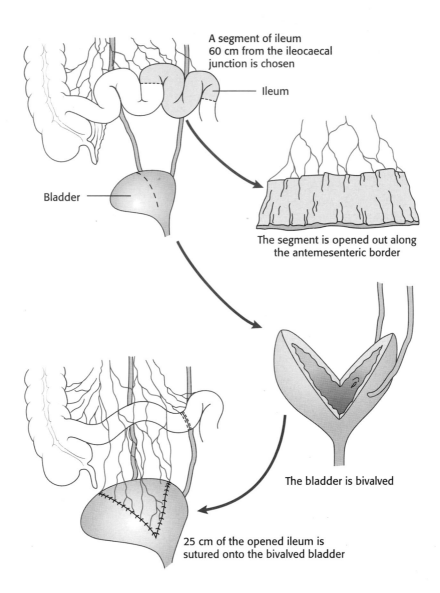

A segment of ileum
60 cm from the ileocaecal
junction is chosen

Ileum

Bladder

The segment is opened out along
the antemesenteric border

The bladder is bivalved

25 cm of the opened ileum is
sutured onto the bivalved bladder

Figure 3.4 Augmentation ileocystoplasty (CLAM) is the most successful surgical
solution to intractable detrusor instability. Double patches are used for the higher
pressure hyperreflexic bladders.

TABLE 3.2

Surgical treatments for detrusor instability

Procedure	Success rate (%)*	Comment
Hydrostatic cystodistension	6	Minimal benefit, but safe
Transtrigonal phenol injection of the pelvic plexus nerves[†]	1 at 12 months	Out of favour
Sacral neurectomy	59	Out of favour
Sacral nerve blockade with phenol	16	Out of favour
Endoscopic bladder transection	16	Out of favour
Detrusor myomectomy	60	Under investigation
Augmentation ileocystoplasty (CLAM)	88	Final treatment

* Defined as cure of incontinence

[†] Serious complications in the form of fistulae have lead to the fall in popularity of this technique

TABLE 3.3

Complications of ileocystoplasty

Complication	Incidence (%)
Early	
Postoperative bleeding	1.5
Ileus	1.9
Wound infection	1.9
Bowel obstruction	3.7
Late	
Mucus in urine (not usually troublesome)	100
Urinary tract infection	34
Malabsorption or acidosis	Non-clinical
Risk of neoplasia	Unknown
Retention requiring long-term CISC	40–100
Cystoplasty rupture	0.9

treat intractable DI have not been particularly successful (Table 3.2) and have not provided any long-term benefit. The only successful surgical solution to intractable DI that is currently available is the CLAM procedure (Figure 3.4).

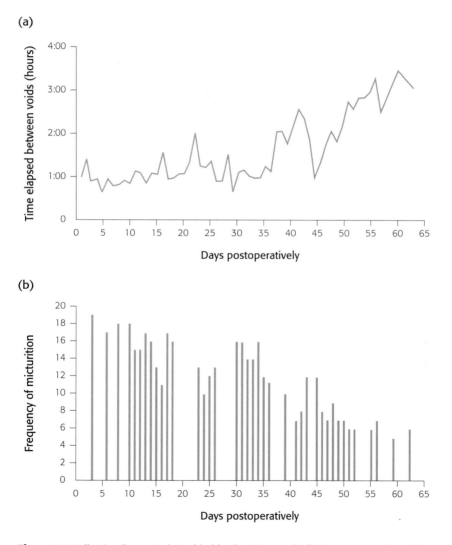

(a)

(b)

Figure 3.5 Following ileocystoplasty, bladder function gradually improves as shown by this carefully recorded diary from a patient postoperatively. (a) The average time elapsing between each void increases and (b) the daily frequency decreases.

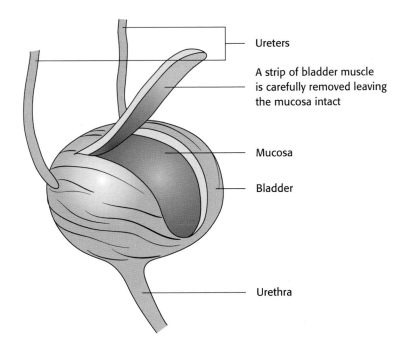

Ureters

A strip of bladder muscle
is carefully removed leaving
the mucosa intact

Mucosa

Bladder

Urethra

Figure 3.6 Detrusor myomectomy.

CLAM provides relief of intractable frequency, urgency and urge incontinence in 90% of patients with idiopathic DI and in 88% of patients with hyperreflexia; these results apply even to elderly patients (Figure 3.5). If a patient is prepared to undergo a major surgical procedure, and is aware of the potential complications (Table 3.3) and the risk (at least 30%) of voiding dysfunction postoperatively necessitating intermittent catheterization, then CLAM may be performed.

More recent modifications of the CLAM procedure using detrusor myomectomy (Figure 3.6), autoaugmentation and demucosalized bowel patches have been developed. Longer term results of the procedures are awaited.

CHAPTER 4
Primary nocturnal enuresis

Primary nocturnal enuresis is defined as urinary incontinence that occurs during sleep in a child who has never 'become dry'. It is a common condition that affects both child and family. Nocturnal enuresis occurs in approximately 20% of children of 5 years of age, 10% of 10-year-olds and 1% of 15-year-olds. In the USA, it is estimated that about 5 million children suffer from the condition.

The fact that the majority of children become dry spontaneously as they grow older should provide some reassurance to both parent and child. However, most parents are concerned that their child becomes dry because of the inconvenience and social stigma that bed-wetting causes.

In 85% of children affected by nocturnal enuresis, daytime urinary habits are normal. However, in children who also suffer daytime symptoms of frequency and urgency, there is a 75% probability of bladder instability.

Aetiology

Nocturnal enuresis can have a number of different aetiologies. Heavy sleeping, in association with either a high fluid intake or the factors associated with nocturnal diuresis, can also cause nocturnal enuresis. Reduced urine osmolality has been shown to be associated with a decreased nocturnal secretion of antidiuretic hormone, giving rise to increased nocturnal urine production. Urine specific gravity is usually less than 1.015 in these circumstances.

The effects of prostaglandin on reducing urethral pressure and increasing detrusor pressure are thought to play a part in some patients. Prostaglandin synthase inhibitors have been used with some success in enuretic patients.

Detrusor instability is most commonly seen in patients who have daytime symptoms of frequency, urgency and urge incontinence. However, 25% of children with primary enuresis with no daytime symptoms may have detrusor instability.

Other factors that may be associated with enuresis are:
- obstruction of the upper airway tract
- a family history (in 65–77% of sufferers).

Primary enuresis has been demonstrated in the presence of a normal bladder capacity, though the capacity may be functionally reduced if instability is present.

Psychological factors have also been extensively investigated and there is disagreement over their contribution. One study concluded that a reduction in self-esteem was a consequence of bed-wetting. Other studies, however, have demonstrated that bed-wetting is not a psychological disorder and no behavioural differences were noted between the bed-wetters and the age-matched control group.

Investigations

It is important to take a comprehensive history of urological symptoms and to ensure that there are no associated abnormalities that require treatment. A physical examination should be carried out, though abnormalities are seldom detected. A measurement of early-morning specific urine gravity may help to diagnose those patients who may benefit from treatment with desmopressin.

It is essential that a urinary diary is kept to demonstrate the extent of the enuresis. A frequency/volume voided chart that shows fluid intake and voided volumes during the day may highlight areas in which simple changes can be made to daily habits, and possibly improve the nocturnal enuresis. A diary of bed-wetting episodes must also be kept to assess the frequency of the problem and to provide a comparison against which the effects of treatment can be measured.

Ultrasound investigation of the kidneys and uroflowmetry is usually only necessary when symptoms suggest urinary tract dysfunction. Urodynamic studies should only be used in those patients with diurnal symptoms who fail to respond to treatment.

Treatment

Many different treatment regimens have been tried for this condition with varying degrees of success. The success rates of the common treatment options are shown in Table 4.1.

The majority of patients 'grow out' of bed-wetting. However, despite assurance that the condition will follow a benign and self-limiting course, many parents and children ask for medical assistance.

TABLE 4.1

The efficacy of treatments for nocturnal enuresis

Treatment	Efficacy
Observation only	6% continent at 6 months;16% at 1 year

Drug therapy

Desmopressin	• Improvement in 79% of patients at 1 year; 50% long-term improvement • 68% continent at 6 months; 10% continent at 1 year • 81% improved by 12 weeks • 48% dry and 22% improved
Amitriptyline	Effective at reducing number of wet nights
Imipramine	36% continent at 6 months; 16% at 1 year; 73% improved

Behavioural interventions

Alarms and sensors	84% dry 63% continent at 6 months; 56% at 1 year
Waking schedule and full-spectrum home training	76% dry
Motivation counselling	23% cure rate (many more helped)
Acupuncture	55% effective at 1 year; 40% long-term improvement
Combination – drugs plus alarms	May produce a complementary benefit

Modifications in fluid intake and output are the simplest means of improving the condition. The use of a diary record may be of benefit, but it is important not to set a high and unattainable goal too early or the child will lose interest. A waking regimen may also be beneficial if the child wets at a particular time of night. Treatment with desmopressin is useful as first- or second-line therapy when alternative measures have failed, or for short-term use when the child is away from home. Treatment should be stopped when the patient becomes dry.

Behavioural therapy and the new 'high-tech' uses of computer-aided biofeedback are useful non-pharmacological treatments. Alarms are used for patients aged 7 years and over, but become most effective after the age of 10 years when the child is able to take responsibility for him- or herself. It is essential that the child is conditioned to wake at the sound of the alarm otherwise it will connect to the sensor and the household, but not the child, will be awoken when the alarm goes off! When the child has been conditioned to the alarm, the sensor and alarm may be used throughout the night.

Up to 7 years of age, anticholinergic drug therapy in the form of imipramine or oxybutynin will be beneficial. Desmopressin will reduce nocturnal urine output and provide dry nights, though this treatment is not recommended for continuous long-term use. The introduction of desmopressin tablets has improved the tolerance of treatment and avoids the side-effects associated with the nasal spray.

By 15 years of age, only 1% of adolescents still suffer from nocturnal enuresis. Each year, a further 15% of these become dry. By this age, urodynamic studies should be performed to check for abnormalities in detrusor function, the commonest of these being DI. Occult neurological dysfunction may be responsible for the enuresis in a small number of patients. In adolescents, drug therapy with anticholinergics is of benefit. After the age of 18 years, patients with persistent enuresis due to detrusor overactivity that does not respond to non-surgical treatment should be offered CLAM (see pages 36–7).

There are some patients who, if enuretic in their teens, are sufficiently psychologically disturbed when all treatment fails to want a surgical solution. The CLAM procedure is very effective in resolving the condition, but counselling is a priority.

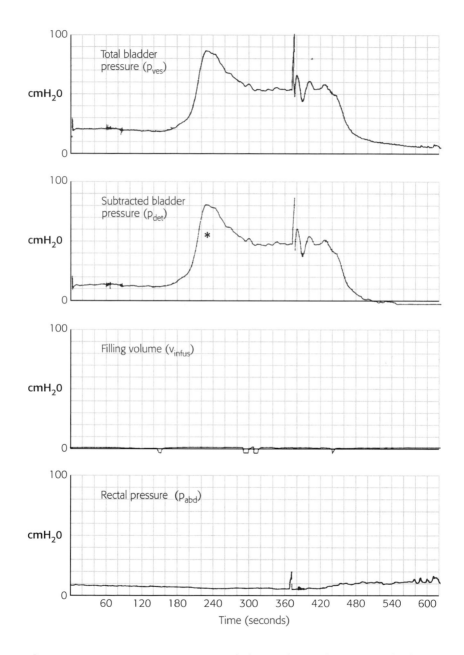

Figure 5.1 Cystometrogram in a patient with detrusor hyperreflexia as a result of a spinal cord injury. ∗, hyperreflexic contraction sustained for 300 seconds.

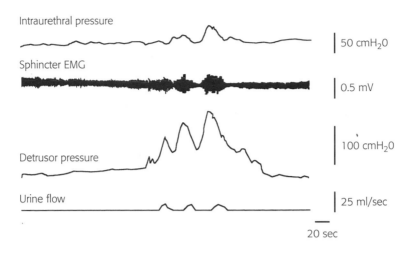

Intraurethral pressure

50 cmH$_2$0

Sphincter EMG

0.5 mV

Detrusor pressure

100 cmH$_2$0

Urine flow

25 ml/sec

20 sec

Figure 5.2 Urodynamic evaluation demonstrating a hyperreflexic detrusor contraction that is fluctuating because of the associated detrusor sphincter dyssynergia.

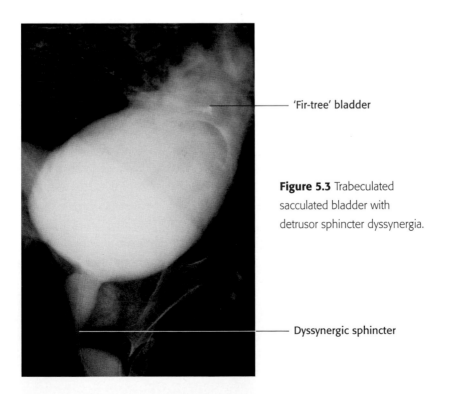

'Fir-tree' bladder

Figure 5.3 Trabeculated sacculated bladder with detrusor sphincter dyssynergia.

Dyssynergic sphincter

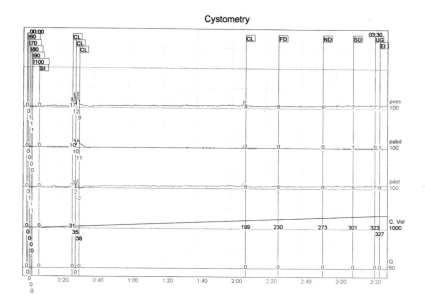

Figure 5.4 Urodynamic evaluation of a patient with acontractile bladder showing no pressure during bladder filling and no emptying pressure. P$_{det}$ (bladder pressure) shows no change during filling and no voiding contraction.

considered and efforts made to uncover an as yet undiagnosed cause, such as multiple sclerosis, a spinal cord lesion or a tethered cord. In suprasacral lesions, neuropathic incontinence is a result of hyperreflexic contractions of the bladder, which are usually associated with the 'urge' type of incontinence, and may be unconscious in those patients with complete lesions affecting the spinal cord. Patients with acontractile bladders tend to leak urine as a result of retention with overflow or in association with sphincter weakness incontinence.

Apart from neurological examination, urodynamic investigation is essential to make an appropriate diagnosis and provide treatment.

Management

An algorithm for the treatment of neuropathic bladder dysfunction is illustrated in Figure 5.5. The aim of management in this disorder is to enable patients to store urine at low pressure and to achieve complete bladder emptying without obstruction. Treatment is therefore aimed at

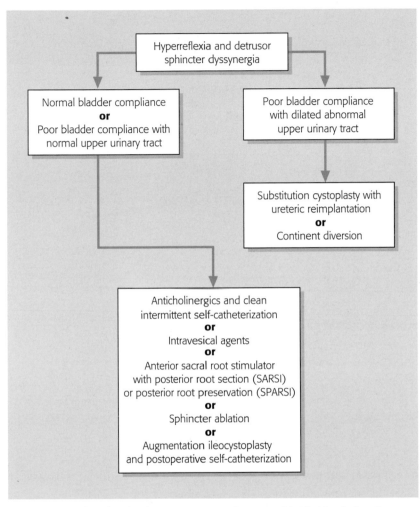

Figure 5.5 An algorithm for the management of neuropathic bladder dysfunction.

either reducing the high-pressure contractions or reducing the effects of DSD by lowering the resistance in the ES. The high-pressure contractions can be controlled either by anticholinergic drugs or by surgery on the detrusor or bladder nerve supply. Although a reduction of the resistance in the ES may be achieved by sphincterotomy or sphincter stenting (Table 5.2), these procedures are appropriate only for those male patients who are willing and able to wear a condom collection device. They are unsuitable for women. A reduction in detrusor hyperreflexia does, however,

TABLE 5.2

Management of detrusor hyperreflexia and detrusor sphincter dyssynergia

To reduce high-pressure detrusor contractions

- Oral anticholinergic medication
- Intravesical anticholinergic medication
- Augmentation ileocystoplasty
- Sacral deafferentation

To reduce or relieve detrusor sphincter dyssynergia

- Anticholinergic medication and intermittent catheterization
- External striated sphincterotomy
- External sphincter stenting
- Permanent suprapubic catheterization
- SARSI

lead to urinary retention; intermittent catheterization is necessary to drain the urine.

Sphincter weakness incontinence, which accompanies neurological bladder dysfunction, may be resolved by procedures to enhance the bladder outlet (see pages 56–62).

Intermittent catheterization

Clean intermittent self-catheterization to empty the bladder usually restores continence in any condition in which the bladder is acontractile and therefore unable to empty, provided there is adequate outlet resistance (Figure 5.6). This technique is used instead of normal bladder emptying on a regular basis throughout the day (and night). The number of catheterizations needed will depend on factors including fluid intake, ambient temperature, bladder capacity and social factors, but most patients should only need to empty the bladder four or five times each day.

The success of intermittent catheterization depends on a number of factors, which include:

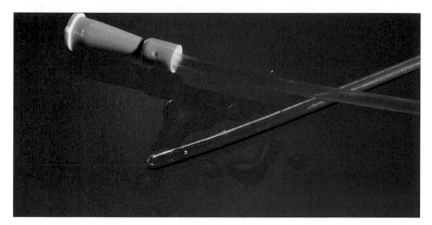

Figure 5.6 Special catheters are available for use in clean intermittent self-catheterization.

- providing a 'stable' bladder that will store urine without leakage through the use of anticholinergic medication
- the type of catheter used (e.g. lubricated)
- the frequency of catheterization
- the accessibility of the urethra (disability may impede access and a caregiver may need to perform the catheterization)
- the ability of health professionals to teach the technique and motivate the patient
- the motivation of the patient.

Long-term catheterization – the suprapubic catheter

Permanent catheterization is normally a last resort when all other treatments have failed. However, it may occasionally be used for shorter periods if patients are undecided as to their preferred management option.

For long-term catheterization, the suprapubic catheter avoids urethral damage, and is more comfortable and more easily tolerated than a catheter inserted via the urethra. It is also easier to change on a regular basis with less discomfort than may be experienced when changing a urethral catheter.

Inserting the suprapubic catheter. Insertion of a suprapubic catheter, preferably for long-term bladder drainage, should be carried out in the operating theatre using endoscopy. The Add-a-Cath® (Bard, UK) is one of

49

the most effective suprapubic catheter insertion systems currently available (Figure 5.7).

Management of the suprapubic catheter. Preservation of normal bladder volume should be achieved by daily distension of the bladder for 1–2 hours by 'catheter clamping' using an in-line valve to the drainage bag.

Drug therapy. Patients with hyperreflexic bladder dysfunction or detrusor instability, such as that seen in multiple sclerosis, spinal cord injury and spina bifida, will also require anticholinergic medication (Table 5.3) If oral therapy cannot be tolerated, intravesical agents such as oxybutynin may be given.

Monitoring. In all patients with spinal cord injury and a permanent suprapubic catheter, the upper urinary tract should be examined every 2 years using ultrasound. This is less essential in other forms of urinary incontinence unless there is an underlying neurological dysfunction, which may give rise to upper urinary tract deterioration if the bladder is not adequately suppressed by anticholinergic medication.

Changing the catheter. The catheter should be changed by an appropriately trained person – a doctor, nurse, care-giver, relative or the patient him/herself. In general, most all-silicone catheters need to be changed every 6–8 weeks.

What if the catheter falls out? Ideally, a catheter should be replaced immediately if it falls out, since the track will start to close very rapidly. After 2 hours, it is usually impossible for a catheter to be reinserted. It is therefore essential that a patient be transferred to hospital immediately if no one is available to insert the new catheter. It is worth giving the patient a catheter to keep at home so that it can easily be inserted if a problem arises.

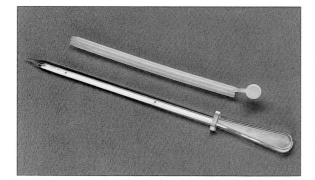

Figure 5.7
Add-a-Cath®: trocar and cannula system for the introduction of a catheter into the bladder via the suprapubic route.

TABLE 5.3

Anticholinergic medication

Agent	Dose
Oxybutynin	2.5 mg three times daily
Propiverine	15.0 mg three times daily
Imipramine	10.0 mg three times daily

What if the catheter blocks frequently? Catheter blockage is a common problem, usually occurring as a result of calcification or debris accumulating within it. Some patients are more prone to blockage than others. If this happens on a regular basis, it is essential that the bladder is checked for calculi or other abnormalities. Some patients who are particularly prone to calcification of their catheters manage in the first instance with a high fluid intake and regular catheter changes. If there is any likelihood of stones or debris within the bladder, an ultrasound scan should be performed and, if necessary, an abdominal radiograph. If the bladder shows signs of calcification, cystoscopy should be performed and any stones removed.

Bladder washouts. Some patients develop blocked catheters because debris in the base of the bladder accumulates in the 'eye' of the catheter when the bladder is empty, or calcification or a biofilm develops along the drainage channel of the catheter.

Instillations and washouts. Antiseptic agents are commonly used, but any proprietary instillation that is squeezed into the bladder tends not to remove any debris lying at the bottom of the bladder. However, an instillation of SubyG® (mandelic acid) will reduce the amount of calcified debris. Turbulent flow within the bladder that enables the debris to be aspirated is necessary to enable removal of debris. Turbulent flow can be achieved by gently inserting 50 ml of sterile saline or boiled tap water into the bladder, and then injecting a further 50 ml more rapidly. Fluid is aspirated rapidly to allow swirling debris to be recovered.

CHAPTER 6

Stress incontinence and mixed incontinence

Genuine stress incontinence is the involuntary loss of urine when intra-abdominal pressure increases during certain activities (see below) and the bladder outlet is weak (sphincter weakness; Table 6.1 and Figure 6.1). This involuntary loss of urine occurs even though the bladder is stable (not contracting). Stress incontinence is associated with a number of different activities; coughing, sneezing, running, jumping, transferring from chair to bed (in paralysed patients), sexual activity and aerobics.

Mixed incontinence is the coexistence of stress incontinence with the urge syndrome. Both men and women may complain of the symptoms of stress incontinence, as well as the symptoms of frequency, nocturia, urgency and urge incontinence, which may or may not be associated with DI.

Approximately 15% of women with mixed incontinence have been shown to have DI on urodynamic testing. If DI is suspected, urodynamic testing is essential. Some patients will have DI that is not diagnosed pre-operatively, but later presents with an exacerbation of symptoms. This applies particularly to women who undergo any form of repositioning

---

TABLE 6.1

Classification of stress incontinence based on X-ray screening

Type 0
A complaint of urinary incontinence but without it being clinically demonstrated

Type I
Urinary incontinence in association with a rise in intra-abdominal pressure in the presence of a normally positioned urethra and bladder neck

Type II
Incompetent bladder neck and hypermobile urethra

Type III
Intrinsic sphincter deficiency – external sphincter weakness in the presence of support to the bladder neck

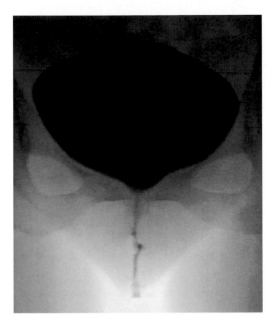

Figure 6.1 Videocystogram showing a combination of bladder base descent and sphincter weakness in a woman with type II stress incontinence.

procedure. Where DI is present, but stress incontinence is the major symptom, anticholinergic medication may resolve the irritative symptoms both before and after surgery if they persist.

Giggle incontinence is a condition that occurs in adolescent girls. The incontinence is commonly described as "I laughed till I wet myself", and is due to a cortically evoked detrusor voiding contraction that produces normal voiding. The condition usually resolves spontaneously as the patient grows up. Medication is of no particular benefit, nor are urodynamic investigations indicated unless there are associated symptoms suggesting bladder dysfunction.

Aetiology

Women. Incontinence in women is due to an intrinsic loss of urethral strength, which is often associated with urethral hypermobility. Childbirth and ageing weaken the urethral sphincter muscles. Childbirth causes denervation of the nerve supply to the pelvic floor and sphincter muscle, and the stretching of the pelvic floor during vaginal delivery will predispose to pelvic floor weakness. Other possible or related causes of stress incontinence in women include obesity, previous pelvic surgery and oestrogen withdrawal related to ageing. Although there is controversy as to the association between obesity and incontinence, the obese patient may prove more difficult to treat because of the increased risk if surgery is to take place.

Stress incontinence in women may also be associated with DI and it is important to identify this during the initial evaluation to ensure that the correct condition is treated appropriately.

Men. Stress incontinence is less common in men because the ES is more powerful and its function does not change significantly with age. In men, incontinence is more likely to develop after prostatic surgery as a result of damage to the ES.

- Transurethral resection of the prostate can result in incontinence, but is unusual (< 1%).
- Incontinence occurs in about 5% of men after retropubic prostatectomy for benign prostatic hyperplasia, but tends to improve with time.
- Approximately 10% of men become incontinent following radical prostatectomy for prostate cancer. This is usually due to a weakness of the external sphincter. However, a combination of DI and loss of bladder compliance may be seen in up to 50% of men with late postoperative incontinence after radical prostatectomy.

Incontinence in men is also commonly caused by DI resulting from prostatic outflow obstruction. An obstructing prostate causes changes in the bladder, giving rise to DI and thus symptoms of frequency, urgency and urge incontinence. Prostatic outflow obstruction may also lead to chronic urine retention and overflow incontinence. Other causes of stress incontinence in men include pelvic fracture, causing damage to the ES, and neurological dysfunction, which occurs in association with spinal cord injury, spina bifida and multiple sclerosis, and may give rise to sphincter weakness.

Diagnosis

Women. The 'clinical diagnosis' of stress incontinence depends on demonstrating the involuntary leakage of urine in the presence of a stable, non-contracting bladder, which is most effectively and accurately shown by urodynamic studies. In the clinic setting, however, stress incontinence may be observed by asking the patient to cough repeatedly (at least six times) with at least 200 ml of urine in the bladder; it is essential that the patient coughs repeatedly, because, in some patients, multiple coughs are necessary to reduce the intra-urethral resistance to the point at which leakage will occur.

Videourodynamic studies are useful because radiological screening enables the bladder neck to be examined (see Figure 6.1, page 53) and the degree to which the bladder base has descended to be assessed. In addition, the ability of the patient to perform a stop-test during mid-flow will provide information about the function of the external urethral sphincter mechanism. If facilities for videourodynamic studies are unavailable, cystometry should be used to exclude associated DI, which may influence subsequent patient management. It should also be remembered that even if urodynamic testing in a patient with both urge and stress incontinence has shown the bladder to be stable, this does not necessarily exclude the presence of DI.

Men. Appropriate urological investigation is recommended in any patient who is sufficiently fit to undergo evaluation and subsequent treatment. The patient should be examined for bladder distension and penile abnormalities, and a digital rectal examination performed to assess the size and consistency of the prostate. A urine culture should always be obtained to exclude infection, which can cause overactivity of the bladder resulting in incontinence. Urinary tract infections in men tend to be associated with a high incidence of urinary tract abnormalities, particularly obstruction.

The simplest investigation in men with voiding dysfunction is flowmetry, together with ultrasound scanning of the bladder to determine the post-micturition residual volume. Ultrasound scanning of the upper urinary tract is useful for highlighting renal abnormalities, particularly dilatation of the renal pelvis and ureters, which is commonly found in association with high-pressure chronic retention. Urodynamic evaluation should be performed in any patient who is sufficiently fit, and certainly in those under the age of 60 years, if surgery is being contemplated. Urodynamic studies should also be performed in patients who have had surgery previously, but are still suffering from incontinence.

Videourodynamic studies, which enable the bladder to be visualized during filling and voiding, are recommended in more complex cases of incontinence, particularly after prostatectomy.

55

In many patients with incontinence following prostatectomy, symptoms will improve over a period of up to 1 year and investigation (flowmetry followed by videourodynamics and cystoscopy) may therefore not be necessary until 6–12 months after surgery.

Medical management in women

A number of therapies are available for the management of stress incontinence (Table 6.2), but the principal medical treatment is pelvic floor strengthening. The muscular activity of the pelvic floor may be improved by:

- performing pelvic floor exercises, either under the supervision of a physiotherapist or continence nurse, or using vaginal cones
- transvaginal electrical stimulation
- use of a perineometer, which measures pelvic floor contractions, and has proved beneficial in some patients.

The simplest treatment to improve pelvic floor strength is to use intra-vaginal cones, which are available commercially, for 15 minutes twice daily. This will improve symptoms in 30% of women with mild stress incontinence. For any of these treatments to be successful, however, the patient must first have sufficient pelvic floor activity to be able to exercise the area, and second be sufficiently motivated to continue with the exercises, because the condition will recur if the patient stops exercising. Thus, for any of these treatments to succeed, professional supervision is important to provide sufficient encouragement and reinforcement. In practice, only relatively minor cases of incontinence will successfully

TABLE 6.2

Non-surgical therapies for stress incontinence in women

- Vaginal cones
- Perineometer
- Pelvic floor electrical stimulation
- Urethral plugs
- Oestrogen replacement
- α-stimulators (phenylpropanolamine)

respond to these techniques, because many patients will stop exercising once reinforcement is removed.

A recent addition to the medical options for urinary incontinence is extracorporeal magnetic innervation (ExMI; Neotonus, Inc., Marietta, GA, USA). The patient sits on a chair that produces pulsed magnetic fields (Figure 6.2). The fields penetrate the perineum, simultaneously stimulating the nerves of the pelvic floor and the sphincter muscles. The physician sets the frequency and strength of the contractions, so that the patient's awareness of their pelvic floor improves, increasing strength in the muscles. Typically, a patient will have two sessions of about 20 minutes a week for 8 weeks or more.

Surgical management in women

It is essential that the cause of the incontinence has been ascertained before surgical treatment is considered. There is no point in subjecting a patient to an operative procedure when the primary cause of the incontinence is unknown, because the procedure may prove worthless.

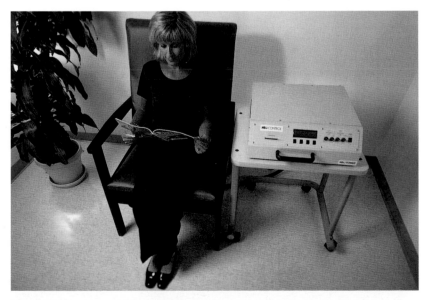

Figure 6.2 In extracorporeal magnetic innervation, a chair that produces pulsed magnetic fields penetrates the perineum, stimulating both the pelvic floor and sphincter nerves. Reproduced with permission from Neotonus, Inc.

The procedure should be selected according to the diagnosis of incontinence based upon the anatomical features. The appropriate procedure will have a higher success rate; although this statement may seem obvious, many patients receive inappropriate treatment, and it is therefore not surprising that treatment may fail. A number of surgical treatments are available (Table 6.3).

Slings are the procedure of choice for patients with ISD as the long-term results are excellent (85% cure rate), and are also often the procedure of choice in women with type II stress incontinence. These procedures are performed by open or minimally invasive surgery.

Tension-free vaginal tape (TVT; Ethicon, Inc., Somerville, NJ, USA) appears to provide good long-term results resulting in a 89% cure rate, and is associated with few complications (Table 6.4). The procedure is minimally invasive, with TVT providing a sling under the urethra without lifting it from its anatomical position (Figure 6.3). Under stress, TVT supports the mid-urethra. Postoperative pain is reduced, and in most cases, patients can return home the same or following day.

Bone anchors provide anchors for sutures in the treatment of female stress incontinence. Through an anterior vaginal wall incision, the bone anchors are placed into the posterior pubic bone with a single-use inserter (Figure 6.4). Sutures attached to the anchors can be used to fix

TABLE 6.3

Surgical procedures for stress incontinence in women

Slings	Open surgical procedures
• Pubo-vaginal sling	• Burch colposuspension
• Autologous slings	• Vagino-obturator shelf procedure
– rectus sheath	**Injectables**
– fascia lata	• Macroplastique® (available in Europe at time of press)
– vaginal wall	
• Artificial suspension (e.g. tension-free vaginal tape, donated and prepared tissues)	• Collagen

TABLE 6.4

Reported complications of tension-free vaginal tape in 17 000 European procedures

Complication	Frequency
Vascular injury	0.00071%
Bowel injury	0.000059%
Bladder perforation	0.7–4.3%
Bleeding	0.32%
Post-operative retention	2.6–6.2%
Wound infection	0.2–1.2%
Erosion	Rare
Death	3 reported in 100 000 cases worldwide

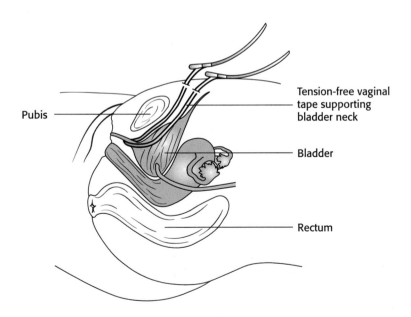

Figure 6.3 Tension-free vaginal tape is positioned close to the urethra, without increasing tension on the vaginal wall. The needles and sleeves are removed when the tape is correctly placed without tension.

periurethral tissues to the pubic bone or to support a sling under the urethra. Postoperative recovery is short and the cure rate high. The long-term results of bone anchors are not yet known.

Open surgical procedures. Burch colposuspension is the most commonly performed open surgical procedure for stress incontinence in which there is at least moderate vaginal mobility (Figure 6.5). This procedure provides good long-term cure for stress incontinence with benefits of 70–80% at 10 years. The use of laparoscopy to assist in this procedure has been investigated, but has been less popular than expected, because of the increased operation time, increased cost and lack of long-term results.

Injection of bulking agents into the urethra is becoming more popular because the procedure is truly 'minimally invasive', involves minimal discomfort and can be performed as an out-patient procedure (Figure 6.6). The results of such treatments vary according to the agent (see Table 6.3) and the technique used, though the long-term benefits

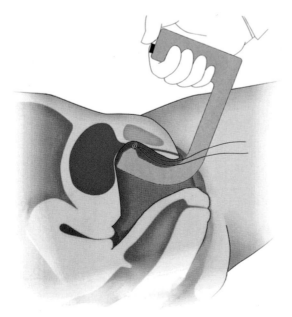

Figure 6.4
Bone anchors are inserted perpendicular to the pubic bone with a single-use applicator.

(a)

Vagina sutured to the
obturator fascia or
pectineal ligament

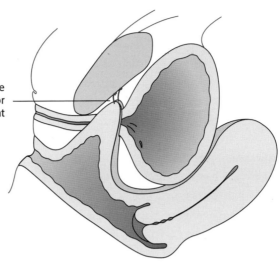

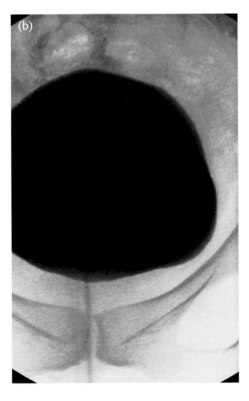

Figure 6.5 (a) In the Burch colposuspension procedure, the vagina is mobilized on either side of the bladder neck and then sutured to the pectineal ligament. This supports the bladder neck and urethra, so that when the patient coughs, the bladder and the urethra do not descend. (b) The X-ray shows a well-supported bladder neck following colposuspension.

(> 5 years) have not yet been reported. If, however, treatment fails, the injection of a bulking agent may be repeated and further open surgery undertaken at a later date. For a woman with a reasonably well-supported bladder neck who remains incontinent, but who wishes to avoid further major surgical procedures, injection of a bulking agent provides an attractive alternative, which can be performed as a relatively painless day-case procedure.

Postoperative complications following surgery for stress incontinence may be subdivided into early and late complications.

Early complications include bleeding and infection, which are relatively uncommon, and voiding dysfunction, which may follow support procedures (occasionally, patients may fail to pass urine or have difficulty in doing so for days or weeks after surgery). Suprapubic catheters are routinely placed after colposuspension to enable assessment of voiding efficiency and to measure residual urine.

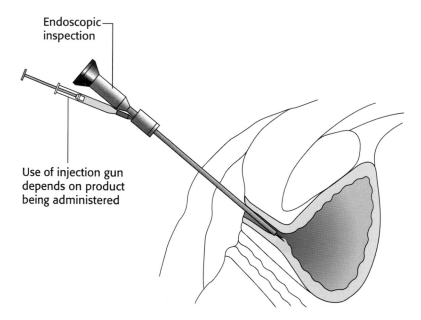

Endoscopic inspection

Use of injection gun depends on product being administered

Figure 6.6 The injected material is placed just beneath the mucosa of the urethra at the level of the bladder neck and proximal urethra, closing the bladder neck and restoring urinary continence.

Late complications include:

- recurrence of stress incontinence, which may be expected in 10–60% of patients (depending upon the technique) within 10 years depending upon the procedure performed
- voiding dysfunction occurs in relatively few patients but may occasionally persist, and necessitate CISC to ensure that the bladder is emptying satisfactorily (in < 2% of patients); pre-operative urodynamics, which demonstrate poor detrusor contractility, provide a warning of potential voiding dysfunction after surgery.

Management in men

Stress incontinence after prostatectomy usually improves spontaneously. Initial management involves strengthening the pelvic floor muscles using pelvic floor exercises. Most patients improve substantially over a period of weeks or months without the need for further investigation or treatment. Any patient who is still suffering from intractable urinary incontinence 6 months after prostatectomy should undergo urodynamic investigation to assess urethral sphincter function. Cystoscopy may also be necessary to ensure that neither a urethral stricture nor any residual prostatic tissue is contributing to the condition. If a clinical and urodynamic diagnosis of sphincter weakness is confirmed and the bladder storage capacity is adequate at low pressure, the treatment options are:

- the use of injectable bulking agents in the sphincter area
- insertion of an artificial urinary sphincter.

Injectable bulking agents are used to treat male stress incontinence; current results are improving because of the adoption of better techniques and the availability of stable injectable materials. Injection into the region of the external sphincter muscle under endoscopy should close the urethra sufficiently to provide continence without affecting bladder emptying.

Artificial urinary sphincter. Insertion of an artificial urinary sphincter (Figure 6.7) is the optimum method of treatment for intractable post-prostatectomy stress incontinence. Provided the bladder pressures are normal during filling, the patient is sufficiently fit to undergo surgery and is able to operate the artificial sphincter. Such treatment should be carried out

63

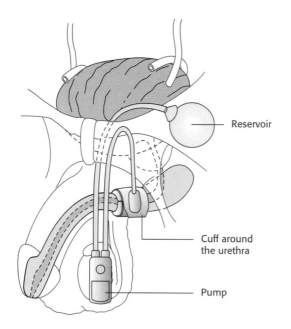

Reservoir

Cuff around
the urethra

Pump

Figure 6.7 The artificial urinary sphincter cuff fits around the bladder neck or urethra and fills with fluid when activated, thereby passively compressing the urethra. To allow voiding, the pump is squeezed two or three times to open the cuff and transfer the fluid to the reservoir. The cuff automatically refills within 1–3 minutes.

at least 1 year after prostatectomy. When the artificial sphincter has been implanted, it is left deactivated for 6 weeks to enable the tissue under the cuff around the urethra to settle, the blood supply to become adequate and for pain at the site of the pump to subside. A capsule is naturally formed around each of the implanted components. During this time, the patient will continue to suffer from incontinence and have to use condom drainage or incontinence pads. When the sphincter is activated, the patient has to learn how to use the sphincter by compressing the pump. The pump should be compressed two or three times to empty the cuff. The cuff will automatically refill from the reservoir within 1–3 minutes.

Complications following insertion of an artificial urinary sphincter are more likely in patients with incontinence caused by neuropathy, exacerbated by high-pressure bladder dysfunction (detrusor hyperreflexia with or without poor bladder compliance; Table 6.5). The most common complications are infection, erosion and mechanical problems. Revision of AMS Sphincter 800™ implantation will be necessary in up to 25% of patients in the first 5 years.

TABLE 6.5

Complications of artificial urinary sphincters

- Erosion
- Infection
- Mechanical dysfunction
- Revision rates increase the longer the implant is present

Elderly patients. Long-term suprapubic catheterization is recommended as an option in elderly patients with dementia. This is because a suprapubic catheter is more comfortable than an indwelling catheter, and is therefore less likely to be pulled out by the patient.

CHAPTER 7
Fistula-related incontinence

Nowadays, urinary incontinence due to the presence of a fistula is fairly uncommon in developed countries – most urologists would expect to see no more than one or two cases a year. However, it is still common in countries in which the level of obstetric care is poor and is due to prolonged or obstructed labour. In developed countries, urinary fistulae are most likely to develop after gynaecological or pelvic surgery, and result from injury to the bladder or ureters (Table 7.1). A fistula develops as a result of the bladder being opened during dissection of the cervix or if the posterior wall of the bladder is inadvertently caught in a suture used for vaginal vault closure. It is important that urinary incontinence due to a fistula is diagnosed as early as possible because further surgery will be necessary to repair the fistula unless the problem can be resolved with minimally invasive techniques. Gynaecological surgery for cancer if complicated by a fistula should indicate the need for biopsy of the fistula site.

Clinical presentation and diagnosis

A patient with a urinary fistula will usually become continuously incontinent in the first few days after a pelvic surgery (Caesarean section or hysterectomy). If the patient was not catheterized during or after surgery, it is important to ensure that urine retention with overflow incontinence is not present. Urine retention can be excluded by palpating the abdomen to see if

---

TABLE 7.1

Types of urinary fistulae

- Vesicovaginal
- Ureterovaginal
- Cervicovaginal and ureterovaginal (after Caesarean section)
- Vesicocutaneous (after suprapubic catheterization) or bladder reconstruction
- Perineal (in association with urethroplasty or urethral strictures)

the bladder is full, or by performing an ultrasound scan of the bladder, which will demonstrate the degree of residual urine. Alternatively, the patient can be catheterized and the residual urine drained and measured. If urine retention is present, the patient should be catheterized as soon as possible to reduce the risk of injury to the bladder muscle caused by over-distension. If the bladder is not full and the patient is voiding leaving no residual urine, it is likely that a fistula has developed. At this stage, the patient should be informed of the possible presence of a fistula and further investigations should be undertaken.

Investigations

Three-swab test. The first investigation that may be performed is a three-swab test, in which three gauze swabs are placed in the vagina and methylene blue injected into the bladder. If the highest swab in the vagina is stained blue, then this is diagnostic of a vesicovaginal fistula (Figure 7.1). If the upper swab is soaked with clear urine, a ureterovaginal fistula is likely. An intravenous urogram should be performed in all women with a suspected fistula.

Cystoscopy is an essential component of the investigation of fistulae. Cystoscopy with simultaneous vaginal examination will reveal the fistulous

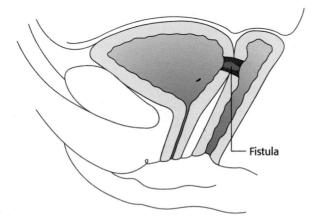

Figure 7.1 Vesicovaginal fistula (bladder/vagina).

site. Instillation of methylene blue into the bladder is valuable when a small vesicovaginal fistula cannot be seen.

Intravenous urogram. If a ureterovaginal fistula is present, contrast leakage at the site of one (or both) of the ureters or pronounced dilatation of one (or both) of the ureters will be seen on the urogram (Figure 7.2) and/or retrograde ureterogram (Figure 7.3).

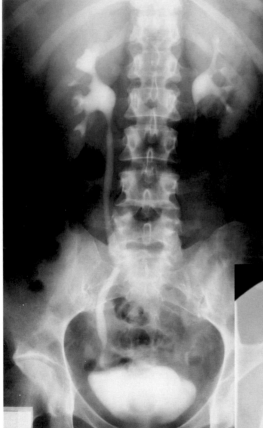

Figure 7.2 Intravenous urogram demonstrating a ureterovaginal fistula.

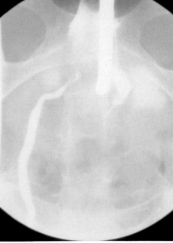

Figure 7.3
Retrograde ureterogram demonstrating right ureteric leakage.

Ureterovaginal fistulae cannot always be confirmed by urography, and cystoscopy and bilateral ureterograms should be performed in all patients in whom they are suspected, and particularly when a vesicovaginal fistula is present. A vesicovaginal fistula may be present along with a ureteric injury.

Treatment

Small vesicovaginal fistulae may heal during a period of continuous catheter drainage, which should be carried out for 2 weeks from the time of first diagnosis.

Ureterovaginal fistulae may resolve if the affected ureter can be stented with a double-J stent, which should be left in place for 6–12 weeks. If conservative management fails, surgery will be necessary.

Ureteric injuries may be operated upon as soon as the diagnosis is confirmed. Vesicovaginal fistulae should be repaired after 3 months when the tissues will be more amenable to surgery.

If it is not possible to insert a ureteric stent or stenting fails to resolve the problem, then treatment should take the form of ureteric reimplantation (Figure 7.4) either by direct implantation into the bladder or by the use of a psoas hitch, Boari flap of bladder or a combination of both procedures. Vesicovaginal fistulae are repaired by open surgery via either the vaginal or the abdominal route. Interposition of healthy tissue in the form of omentum,

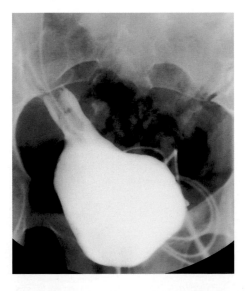

Figure 7.4 Radiograph demonstrating ureteric implantation with psoas hitch.

if performed abdominally, or as a Martius graft, if performed vaginally, between the vagina and bladder greatly enhances the success of the procedure.

CHAPTER 8
Urinary diversion

Most patients can be cured of their incontinence by using one or several of the procedures described in the preceding chapters. There will always be a few patients, however, who remain incontinent. Urinary diversion may be contemplated in these patients provided they are sufficiently motivated to become continent again, or the patient is so debilitated (e.g. in advanced multiple sclerosis) that a urinary diversion is a last resort. Surface diversion leaving the bladder *in situ* may also be performed (Figure 8.1).

The simplest diversion is a catheter, preferably the long-term all-silicone suprapubic catheter (see Chapter 5). However, for patients who wish to avoid long-term catheterization, those in whom outlet resistance is very poor, and those who wish to have greater control of 'bladder emptying', reconstructive diversion should be considered after appropriate counselling.

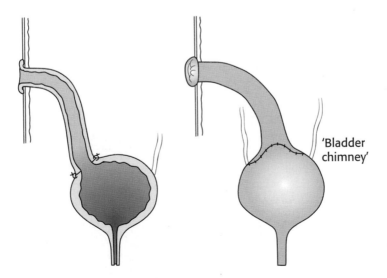

'Bladder chimney'

Figure 8.1 Surface diversion leaving the bladder *in situ*. The bladder is connected to the skin surface by a conduit of ileum. This provides the benefit of urinary diversion without the need to remove the bladder and leaves the ureters attached to their normal position in the bladder.

Ureterosigmoidostomy

Ureterosigmoidostomy has been in use for more than 100 years (Figure 8.2). The ureters are implanted into the sigmoid colon, and both urine and faeces are passed via the rectum. The procedure is not commonly performed in the west, but is still used in occasional patients. A modification of this technique, in which a larger pouch of sigmoid is created for the storage of urine (the Mainz II pouch; Figure 8.3) has recently become more popular. The ureterosigmoidostomy, which avoids the need for a 'bag', may be associated with hyperchloraemic acidosis. Cancer formation at the site of the junction of the ureter with bowel is 30 times more common than normal, and annual inspection of the junction by colonoscopy is necessary from 5 years after the procedure.

Bladder neck/urethral closure and long-term catheterization

In the very disabled patient with complete urethral incompetence due to long-term indwelling catheterization, bladder neck closure and a surgically

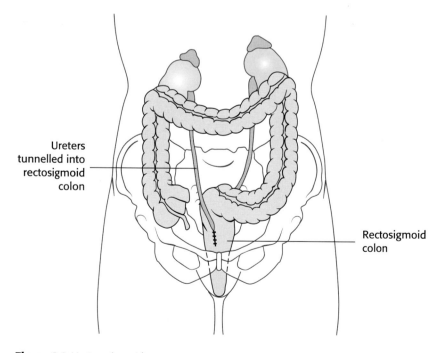

Ureters tunnelled into rectosigmoid colon

Rectosigmoid colon

Figure 8.2 Ureterosigmoidostomy.

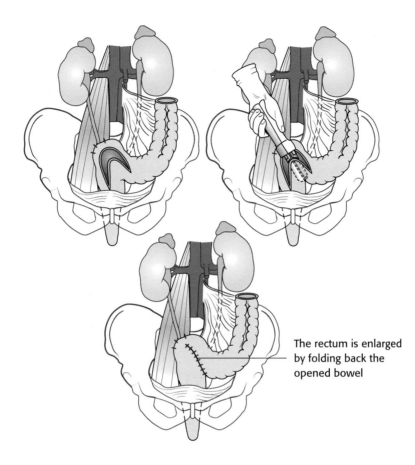

The rectum is enlarged by folding back the opened bowel

Figure 8.3 Mainz II pouch procedure.

implanted suprapubic catheter are very effective. Urethral/bladder neck closure may be accomplished via a vaginal approach with minimal morbidity. This procedure may be combined with the Mitrofanoff principle (see page 75) instead of a long-term catheter.

Surface diversion

Ileal conduit urinary diversion (Figure 8.4) has provided effective urinary tract drainage for many patients in the 35 years since it was first introduced. Although it is a major procedure, it is also relatively straightforward. Complications arising from the procedure are similar to those seen after

73

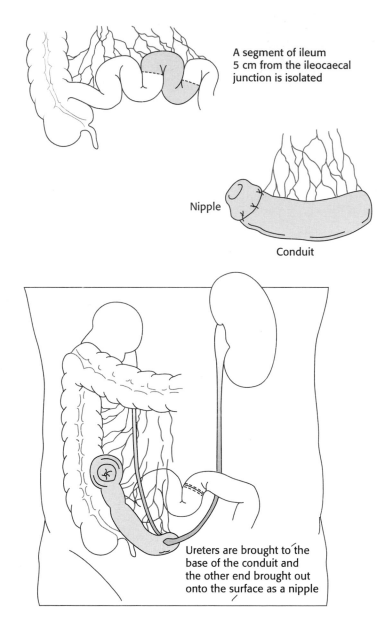

A segment of ileum
5 cm from the ileocaecal
junction is isolated

Nipple

Conduit

Ureters are brought to the
base of the conduit and
the other end brought out
onto the surface as a nipple

Figure 8.4 Ileal conduit urinary diversion involves disconnecting the ureters from the
bladder and attaching them to a segment of ileum, which is brought out at a suitable
site as a surface stoma. A collecting appliance is placed on the abdominal skin surface
to allow collection of urine.

TABLE 8.1

Late complications of surface urinary diversion

- Intestinal obstruction
- Urinary tract infection
- Stomal prolapse and/or obstruction
- Metabolic acidosis
- Urinary tract stone disease
- Upper tract deterioration with reflux and hydronephrosis

surgery to the abdomen (Table 8.1). Upper tract deterioration may occur many years after urinary diversion and thus careful long-term follow up is recommended. If properly counselled, most patients are content with their urinary diversion if the preceding urinary incontinence has been particularly troublesome and if many surgical procedures have failed.

Continent diversion

Providing a continent catheterizable reservoir for the storage of urine is an attractive option, particularly for younger patients who are intractably incontinent and wish to avoid surface urinary diversion. Many procedures are available for continent diversion, all of which involve modifications of the principle described by Koch (Figure 8.5) or Studer. The remaining bladder may be used as a base for bowel reconstruction, or a neobladder may be created from bowel segments. The patient is then able to catheterize the bowel pouch through a connection from the abdominal wall. This connection may be made via a continent port made from tailored bowel, or via the appendix which, in turn is tunnelled into the pouch (Mitrofanoff principle; Figure 8.6). Continent diversion involves more intricate and time-consuming surgery than surface diversion, and thus is associated with a slightly greater risk of early complications (Table 8.2).

Mitrofanoff with Monti procedure

One or two segments of ileum are chosen for the catheterization tube (Figure 8.6a). The segment(s) is isolated from the bowel continuity. The

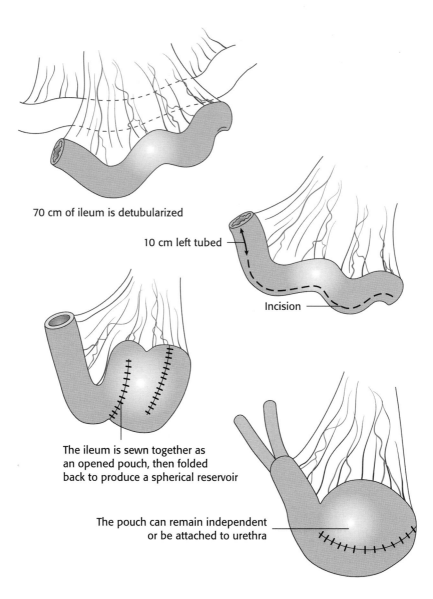

70 cm of ileum is detubularized

10 cm left tubed

Incision

The ileum is sewn together as
an opened pouch, then folded
back to produce a spherical reservoir

The pouch can remain independent
or be attached to urethra

Figure 8.5 If a patient does not wish to have a surface diversion, an internal diversion
may be created. The procedure involves the formation of a neobladder or pouch from
a section of intestine, usually the ileum. The reservoir is connected to the abdominal
skin surface by the appendix or a tube of intestine which is tunnelled into the pouch
providing a continence mechanism.

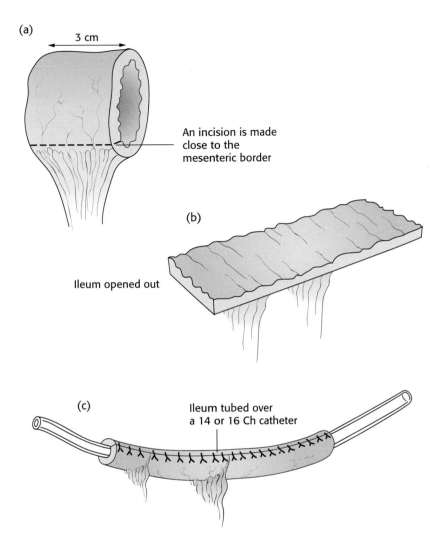

(a) 3 cm

An incision is made close to the mesenteric border

(b)

Ileum opened out

(c) Ileum tubed over a 14 or 16 Ch catheter

Figure 8.6 The Mitrofanoff principle with Monti procedure. (a) A segment of ileum is chosen for the catheterization tube and isolated from the bowel continuity. (b) The bowel is divided close to the mesentery and the ileum opened out. (c) The ileum is then tubed over a 14 or 16 Ch catheter. The tube can then be tunnelled into the bladder or neobladder and attached to a skin opening.

bowel is divided close to the mesentery and the ileum opened out. The ileum is then tubed over a 14 or 16 Ch catheter. The tube can be tunnelled into the

TABLE 8.2

Complications of continent urinary diversion

- Death (< 1%)
- Stomal stenosis
- Catheterization difficulties
- Prolapse of the continent nipple
- Pouch stone formation
- Urinary leakage from pouch
- Metabolic complications
- Excess mucus production
- Urinary infection
- Pouch rupture
- Reflux
- Upper tract deterioration

bladder or neobladder and attached to a skin opening. Two tubes, end to end, can be used to bridge a longer distance.

CHAPTER 9
Future trends

Urinary incontinence is a common clinical problem which, if approached in a systematic manner, can be cured in most, if not all, patients. In the future, as patients become more aware that urinary incontinence can be treated, the demand for patient care in this area will increase. This increase in demand for treatment will have to be met by a redistribution of resources and it may act as the necessary driving force to encourage more and better training in this specialist field. The increase in demand for treatment of urinary incontinence will affect all health professionals and in particular the family physician who is the first port of call for the troubled patient. Rapid advances in the field of incontinence therapy must be communicated to those involved with treatment.

In the future, more importance should be placed on the accurate determination of subjective and objective long-term results of treatment for incontinence. Furthermore, better methods of evaluating the improvement in quality of life following various treatments need to be developed and the results balanced against the cost of the treatment.

Conservative management

The incidence of urinary incontinence could be reduced in the future by a number of conservative measures:

- by increasing patient awareness about the benefits of performing pelvic floor exercises, not only before and after childbirth, but throughout life along with the other general improvements in lifestyle
- through improvements in the design and cost of devices for stimulating pelvic floor muscular activity
- through improved standards of obstetric care in developing countries.

Surgical management

Advances in surgical techniques are being made, with more effective bladder neck suspension procedures being developed and less invasive methods of performing sling procedures being devised. Intra-urethral devices for the treatment of urinary incontinence in women are still experimental and expensive. If such devices can be made small enough to fit comfortably without causing urethral injury, then intra-urethral devices may prove to be beneficial in women who wish to avoid surgery. Experimental work is also under way to improve the artificial urinary sphincter.

The most effective surgical procedures for stress urinary incontinence are the open suspension and sling procedures. The less invasive needle suspension procedures have now almost disappeared and day-case sling procedures are becoming the norm. Despite the large number of surgical procedures available for treating urinary incontinence, some women suffer a recurrence of incontinence following a single procedure, though may become dry after a combination of procedures or successive procedures. The ideal is to proceed to more effective procedures (i.e. sling procedures) immediately.

Curing all cases of urinary incontinence, the ideal for all patients, remains an obvious challenge, which will have rewards for both patient and clinician.

Key references

GENERAL

Leach G, ed. *Atlas Of The Urologic Clinics Of North America: Vaginal Surgery For The Urologist*. Philadelphia: WB Saunders, 1994.

EVALUATION OF FEMALE INCONTINENCE

Blaivas JG, Olsson CA. Stress incontinence: classification and surgical approach. *J Urol* 1988;139:727–31.

Griffiths D. Clinical aspects of detrusor instability and the value of urodynamics: a review of the evidence. *Eur Urol* 1998; 34(Suppl 1):13–15.

Hampel C, Weinhold D, Benken N *et al*. Prevalence and natural history of female incontinence. *Eur Urol* 1997; 32(Suppl 2):3–12.

Massey A, Abrams P. Urodynamics of the female lower urinary tract. *Urol Clin N Am* 1985;12:231–46.

McGuire E. Urodynamic evaluation of stress incontinence. *Urol Clin N Am* 1995; 22:551–5.

Steele AC, Kohli N, Mallipeddi P, Karram M. Pharmacologic causes of female incontinence. *Int Urogynecol J Pelvic Floor Dysfunct* 1999;10:106–10.

Zimmern PE. The role of voiding cystourethrography in the evaluation of the female lower urinary tract. *Prob Urol* 1991;5:23–41.

MANAGEMENT OF TYPICAL STRESS INCONTINENCE

Black NA, Downs SH. The effectiveness of surgery for stress incontinence. *Br J Urol* 1996;78:497–510.

Burch JC. Urethrovaginal fixation to Cooper's ligament for correction of stress incontinence, cystocele, and prolapse. *Am J Obstet Gynecol* 1961;81:281–90.

Cardozo L. Role of estrogens in the treatment of female urinary incontinence. *J Am Ger Soc* 1990;38:326–8.

Cardozo L, Hextall A, Bailey J, Boos K. Colposuspension after previous failed incontinence surgery: a prospective observational study. *Br J Obstet Gynaecol* 1999;106:340–4.

Habb F, Leach GE. Feasibility of outpatient percutaneous bladder neck suspension under local anesthesia. *Urology* 1997;50:585–7.

Habb F, Trockman BA, Zimmern PE *et al*. Quality of life and continence assessment of the artificial urinary sphincter in men with minimum 3.5 years of follow-up. *J Urol* 1997;158:435–9.

Hahn I, Sommar S, Fall M. A comparative study of pelvic floor training and electrical stimulation for the treatment of genuine female stress urinary incontinence. *Physiotherapy* 1991;77:545–54.

Jarvis GJ. Surgery for genuine stress incontinence. *Br J Gynaecol* 1994;101: 371–4.

Kegel AH. Progressive resistance exercise in the functional restoration of the perineal muscles. *Am J Obstet Gynecol* 1948; 56:238–48.

Kelly MJ, Leach GE. Long-term results of bladder neck suspension procedures. *Urology* 1991;37:213.

Lawton V, Smith AR. Laparoscopic colposuspension. *Semin Laparosc Surg* 1999;6:90–9.

Leach GL, Dmochowski RR, Appell RA *et al*. Female stress urinary incontinence clinical guidelines panel summary report on surgical management in female stress urinary incontinence. *J Urol* 1997; 158:875–80.

Marshall VF, Marchetti AA, Krantz KE. The correction of stress incontinence by simple vesicourethral suspension. *Surg Gynecol Obstet* 1949;88:509–18.

Olsson I, Kroon U. A three-year postoperative evaluation of tension-free vaginal tape. *Gynecol Obstet Invest* 1999;48:267–9.

Ross J. Laparoscopy or open Burch colposuspension? *Curr Opin Obstet Gynecol* 1998;10:405–9.

Sheriff MK, Foley S, Mcfarlane J *et al*. Endoscopic correction of intractable stress incontinence with silicone micro-implants. *Eur Urol* 1997;32:284–8.

Stamey TA. Endoscopic suspension of the vesical neck for urinary incontinence. *Surg Gynecol Obstet* 1973;136:547–54.

Stanton SL, Hilton P, Norton C *et al*. Clinical and urodynamic effects of anterior colporrhaphy and vaginal hysterectomy for prolapse with and without incontinence. *Br J Obstet Gynaecol* 1982;89:459–63.

Ulmsten U, Falconer C, Johnson P *et al*. A multicenter study of tension-free vaginal tape (TVT) for surgical treatment of stress urinary incontinence. *Int Urogynecol J Pelvic Floor Dysfunct* 1998;9:210–13.

Ulmsten U, Johnson P, Rezapour M. A three-year follow up of tension free vaginal tape for surgical treatment of female stress urinary incontinence. *Br J Obstet Gynaecol* 1999;106:345–50.

Wang AC, Lo TS. Tension-free vaginal tape. A minimally invasive solution to stress urinary incontinence in women. *J Reprod Med* 1998;43:429–34.

TREATMENT OF INTRINSIC SPHINCTERIC DEFICIENCY

Amundsen C, Lau M, English SF, McGuire EJ. Do urinary symptoms correlate with urodynamic findings? *J Urol* 1999; 161:1871–4.

Chaikin DC, Rosenthal J, Blaivas JG. Pubovaginal fascial sling for all types of stress urinary incontinence: long-term analysis. *J Urol* 1998;160:1312–16.

Conrad S, Pieper A, de la Maza SF *et al*. Long-term results of the Stamey bladder neck suspension procedure: a patient questionnaire based outcome analysis. *J Urol* 1997;157:1672–7.

Cross CA, Cespedes RD, McGuire EJ. Our experience with pubovaginal slings in patients with stress urinary incontinence. *J Urol* 1998;159:1195–8.

Cross CA, English SF, Cespedes RD, McGuire EJ. A follow up on transurethral collagen injection therapy for urinary incontinence. *J Urol* 1998;159:106–8.

Cummings JM. Leakpoint pressures in female stress urinary incontinence. *Int Urogynecol J Pelvic Floor Dysfunct* 1997;8:153–5.

Haab F, Zimmern PE, Leach GE. Urinary stress incontinence due to intrinsic sphincteric deficiency: experience with fat and collagen periurethral injections. *J Urol* 1997;157:1283–6.

Pycha A, Klingler CH, Haitel A *et al.* Implantable microballoons: an attractive alternative in the management of intrinsic sphincter deficiency. *Eur Urol* 1998;33: 469–75.

Romanzi LJ, Chaikin DC, Blaivas JG. The effect of genital prolapse on voiding. *J Urol* 1999;161:581–6.

MANAGEMENT OF CYSTOCELE AND PELVIC PROLAPSE

Dmochowski RR, Zimmern PE, Ganabathi K *et al.* Role of the four-corner bladder neck suspension to correct stress incontinence with a mild to moderate cystocele. *Urology* 1997;49:35–40.

Hoffman MS, Harris MS, Bouis PJ. Sacrospinous colpopexy in the management of uterovaginal prolapse. *J Reprod Med* 1996;41:299–303.

Viera AJ, Larkins-Pettigrew M. Practical use of the pessary. *Am Fam Physician* 2000;61:2719–26, 2729.

Zimmern PE, Leach GE, Ganabathi K. The urological aspects of vaginal wall prolapse. Part I: diagnosis and surgical indications. Part II: surgical techniques, complications and results. *AUA Update Series* 1993;XII:25–6.

Now test yourself...

You've read the book, so why not visit

www.fastfactsbooks.com

to test your new-found knowledge on urinary continence. You'll find 20 questions designed to ensure that you have picked up the key points on managing this distressing condition.

Index